Acknowledgments

To the army of counsellors that have worked with The Listening Post C.I.C having a shared passion to provide counselling to those who have needed our support.

To those that have continued to support The Listening Post C.I.C since its inception and continue to help us raise money, spread the word and offer different expertise, we are always grateful.

To our past, present, and future clients, thank you for placing your trust in us and allowing us the privilege to walk your ~~th with you.

About the Author

The Listening Post C.I.C is a not-for-profit Counselling agency set up in 2016, with the aim of breaking the stigma around mental health and provide support as people needed it, breaking the barriers that prevent many people from accessing support with their mental health.

We truly believe that everyone has the right to be heard and listened to without fear and judgement. Facilitating opportunities to make changes for themselves that will enable them to live their best possible lives.

The Listening Post C.I.C

Community Counselling Service

The Invisible Fight

Overcoming Anxiety

Table of Contents

Dedication

This book is dedicated to all those that fight the invisible fight on a daily basis.

Keep up the fight as you're worth it.

Introduction

Life is a series of seasons, some good while others are overwhelming and debilitating. One thing all seasons have in common is a whirlwind of emotions. At some point in our lives, we will face emotions that hold a tight grip on our minds and state of being. But one of the most intense feelings that we can experience is anxiety.

Anxiety is a normal part of life, but it can be debilitating when it becomes overwhelming and begins to interfere with daily activities. Anxiety disorders affect millions of people worldwide, ranging from mild to severe. Fortunately, there are effective coping mechanisms that can help manage anxiety and prevent it from taking over one's life.

In this book, we will explore the importance of learning to cope with anxiety and provide you with practical strategies and techniques that you can use to manage your symptoms. We will cover the symptoms, root causes, and how they can impact your life. We will also discuss ways to respond to anxiety to help you regain control when feeling out of control.

It is essential to understand that anxiety is a natural stress response, but it can become problematic when it becomes chronic and disruptive. If left untreated, anxiety can lead to physical health problems, depression, and other mental health disorders. Coping with anxiety is essential to maintaining good mental health and overall well-being.

Throughout this book, we will provide you with tools and techniques that you can use to manage your anxiety symptoms. These strategies include mindfulness, relaxation techniques, and cognitive-behavioral therapy. We will also discuss the importance of self-care and developing a support system to help you manage your anxiety.

When we get knocked down, how we respond dictates what comes next, how we feel, and what comes out of the situation. In this guide, we will provide you with the knowledge and tools to help you manage anxiety so you can be empowered to take the driver's seat of your emotions and thrive in all areas of life!

Let's get started!

Chapter 1 | Developing Mindfulness

Distractions are everywhere around us. Constantly our attention is being pulled into multiple directions, whether related to work, children, family life, friends, or commitments. The reality is that we live amid busyness—which can cause *stress* and *anxiety*. And add to that the challenges we face in different areas of our lives, whether it's marital struggles, financial crises, relationship issues, and problems at work, among others.

It becomes much more difficult to take a step back and be retrospective. So, what can we do? We develop *mindfulness*. Mindfulness involves cultivating awareness and attention to the present moment without judgment or distraction. When you become self-aware, you begin to notice tendencies. You become in tune with your thought-life, and you sense patterns. These patterns can leave a trail as to what thoughts are responsible for the anxiety you experience.

When you pay attention to your thoughts, you will identify two tendencies.

1. Focus: The mind focuses on things other than what is happening now.

2. Evaluation: The mind continuously evaluates our reality as good or bad.

These tendencies are part of the human experience. And quite frankly, they are inevitable. We either think about the past, the present, or the future. Thinking about the past is backward thinking, and thinking about the future is forward thinking. Both can cause *anxiety*. We may dive into negative emotions of regret and pain when we think about our past. And when we think about the future, we may feel fear and anxiety because it's unknown. We may even think about adverse outcomes or all the bad turns our life can take.

But something disrupts these tendencies—focusing on the present. When we focus on our present, we eliminate the automatic effort to judge things in the past or future. Mindfulness is the anecdote to shift our focus from the past and future onto what's happening at the moment. Interestingly, mindfulness is much more than acknowledging the present. It's about diving deeper and being intentional. It's about cultivating a connection with our present experience.

Here are some strategies for developing mindfulness to help you cope with anxiety:

1. Practice mindfulness meditation: One of the most effective ways to cultivate mindfulness is through regular meditation. Mindfulness meditation involves focusing on the present moment, such as your breath or bodily sensations, and noticing when your mind wanders without judgment.

2. Pay attention to your senses: Another way to become more conscious is to focus your attention on your senses. For example, when you're eating, pay attention to your food's taste, texture, and aroma. When you're outside, notice the sights, sounds, and smells around you. When you are becoming anxious, think about your thoughts and what fear-induced thoughts are causing the anxiety to rise.

3. Take breaks from technology: Technology can be a major distraction that pulls us away from the present moment. To become more conscious, try taking breaks from technology, such as turning off your phone or computer for a few hours each day.

4. Practice gratitude: Focusing on what you're grateful for can help you become more conscious of the positive aspects of your life. Take time each day to reflect on what you're thankful for—a supportive friend, a beautiful sunset, or a favorite hobby. Gratitude decreases anxiety helping your focus on the good around you.

5. Engage in mindful activities: Engaging in activities that require focused attention, such as yoga, tai chi, or painting, can help you develop mindfulness. It will relax you when you feel nervous or anxious about something in your life.

6. Be present with others: When you're with other people, try to be fully present and engaged in the conversation. Avoid distractions such as phones or other devices, and focus on actively listening and responding to the person in front of you.

As you develop mindfulness, you can uncover the root cause of your anxiety and what thoughts trigger it. Once you can identify the source of your anxiety, then you can learn to respond to it.

"You cannot treat what you cannot see."

Chapter 2 | Practical Exercises and CBT

You can learn to help yourself despite the magnitude of what you face. You must look within, understand yourself, and identify your particular needs. The truth is that thoughts, feelings, and behaviors are connected. They work together in an upward or downward spiral. When you are experiencing a low mood, it will affect your level of motivation, and you will find it challenging to be creative and enjoy things in life.

As our mood continues downward and becomes obscured by negative thoughts that cause worry and fear, they will likely lead us to freeze. In other words, you become paralyzed emotionally. Thus, affecting your ability to respond appropriately. So, what happens? Our anxiety can interfere with our daily life. We pull back from work, we become irritable, stress takes over, and we may isolate ourselves—which can lead to depression because we feel hopeless.

When this happens, the following are three things you can do are:

1. Practice deep breathing and relaxation techniques, such as progressive muscle relaxation or guided meditation, to help calm the body and mind.

2. Challenge negative thoughts and replace them with more realistic or positive ones using cognitive restructuring.

3. Engage in physical activity or hobbies that help distract from anxious thoughts and promote relaxation, such as walking, reading a book, or practicing a creative outlet like painting or writing.

Breathing and Relaxation

One breathing technique that someone can practice when feeling anxious is the 4-7-8 breathing technique.

To practice this technique, you should:

1. Sit or lie down in a comfortable position.

2. Close your eyes and take a deep breath in through your nose for 4 seconds.

3. Hold your breath for 7 seconds.

4. Exhale slowly through your mouth for 8 seconds, making a whooshing sound.

5. Repeat this cycle 4-5 times or until you feel calmer.

This technique can help slow down your breathing, increase oxygen flow to the brain, and activate the body's relaxation response, decreasing anxiety and promoting relaxation.

Challenge Negative Thoughts

Did you know that negative thinking is a habit? It's a habit we must break and transform, and you can do so by challenging your negative thoughts through cognitive restructuring.

Challenge negative thoughts with the following steps:

1. Identify the negative thought: Pay attention to the thoughts that come up when you are feeling anxious

and identify the negative or unrealistic thoughts contributing to your anxiety.

2. Question the evidence: Ask yourself if any evidence supports this negative thought. Are there any facts or information that contradict it?

3. Challenge the thought: Consider alternative explanations or interpretations of the situation that could be more realistic and balanced. Ask yourself if there are other ways to view the less negative or catastrophic situation.

4. Replace with a positive thought: Replace the negative thought with a more positive and realistic one. For example, if the negative thought was "I won't be able to do it," replace it with "I'm capable and can do all things."

Engage with Activities

When anxiety starts creeping up, you can automatically respond by engaging with life, activities, or people that boost your mood. These activities can be hobbies you enjoy, conversations that encourage you, or make you laugh. Spending time with people that make you feel good is essential, so associations can be a great source of support. Doing something positive not only lifts your mood but also boosts your perspective, helping you replace negative thoughts with positive ones.

Cognitive Behavioral Therapy

The practices mentioned above have been proven helpful throughout many studies. These practical strategies are also part of CBT or Cognitive Behavioral Therapy. CBT is a form of psychological therapy that focuses on changing negative thought patterns and behaviors to improve emotional and mental well-being.

The following are four aspects of CBT:

1. **Focus on the present**: It's a present-focused therapy that aims to help individuals manage their current problems and symptoms. It is less concerned with exploring the past and more focused on teaching skills to help individuals cope with current challenges.

2. **Collaboration between therapist and client**: CBT is a collaborative process between the therapist and the client. The therapist works with the client to identify negative thought patterns and behaviors and teaches them coping skills and techniques to challenge and modify them.

3. **Cognitive restructuring**: A core aspect of CBT involves cognitive restructuring, which involves identifying and changing negative thought patterns and beliefs. The therapist helps the client identify automatic negative thoughts and teaches them how to challenge and replace them with more positive, realistic thoughts.

4. **Behavioral activation**: CBT also focuses on changing negative behaviors and increasing positive behaviors. The therapist works with the client to identify behaviors that reinforce negative thoughts and emotions and helps them develop strategies to engage in more positive and fulfilling activities.

There are five areas of Cognitive Behavioral Therapy: thoughts, behaviors, emotions, physical sensations, and environments. In other words, your entire human experience can be impacted by anxiety—your thoughts, actions, your health, and the people around you. Overall, CBT can help improve your overall quality of life so that you can decrease stress and form more positive mental pathways.

Life is hard, but we can make the best out of tough situations and challenging emotions with two things— knowledge and application. Now that you know how to respond to anxiety to breathe, challenge your thoughts, and engage in activities, we can navigate the depths of our thought-life.

Chapter 3 | Thought-Life

Beyond the problems we face and our negative thoughts, we overlook the mental loops we engage in because they have become normal. But just because they seem normal does not mean they should not be challenged and changed. First, think about what your thoughts look like daily. What do you think about most? What worries you about your life right now? What keeps you up at night?

Let's identify a few negative thoughts that may emerge daily:

1. "I'm not good enough" - this can relate to working, personal relationships, or even physical appearance.

2. "Things will never get better" - this thought may arise you are going through a difficult time or facing an insurmountable challenge.

3. "Nobody cares about me" - this thought may arise when you feel neglected or unsupported by those around you.

4. "I'll never be able to do it" - this thought can come up when you are facing a new challenge or learning something new, and you doubt your ability to succeed.

5. "I'm a failure" – you can think this when you experience a setback or disappointment and feel like you've let yourself or others down.

6. "Nothing ever goes my way" - this thought can arise when you feel like you're constantly facing obstacles and setbacks, and you feel like you can't catch a break.

7. "I don't deserve happiness" – this thought is a sign of low self-esteem or when you feel like you've done something to warrant unhappiness in your life.

These are just a few examples, and what they all have in common is that they cause you to experience anxiety because they all lead to catastrophizing, racing thoughts, and frustration.

Catastrophizing

Negative thoughts can lead to catastrophizing because they trigger the brain's "fight or flight" response, causing us to perceive threats as much bigger and more dangerous than they actually are. This can create a cycle of negative thoughts that reinforce and amplify one another, leading to an exaggerated sense of danger and a heightened emotional response.

The best approach to catastrophizing is to begin your breathing exercise mentioned in chapter two and then put things into perspective. You've already thought about all the possible ways things can go wrong. Stop yourself immediately and start thinking about all the possible ways things can go in your favor.

Here are seven things you can say to yourself when you are catastrophizing over a situation:

1. "What evidence do I have to support this catastrophic thinking?"

Evaluate the situation more objectively and consider alternative, more balanced perspectives.

2. "Is this thought helpful or productive?"

Question the usefulness of your catastrophic thinking and redirect your focus toward more constructive thoughts.

3. "What's the worst that could happen, and how likely is it to occur?"

Evaluate the realistic risks associated with the situation.

4. "How can I prepare for or prevent the worst-case scenario?"

Focus on problem-solving and taking proactive steps to address potential risks or challenges.

5. "What positive outcomes or opportunities could arise from this situation?"

Focus on potential benefits or opportunities that could emerge from the situation rather than just dwelling on the negative.

6. "What have I done in similar situations before, and what did I learn from those experiences?"

Draw on past experiences and use them to inform your current approach.

7. "What would I say to a friend or loved one if they were going through this situation?"

Adopt a more compassionate and supportive perspective toward yourself, which can help reduce feelings of anxiety or distress.

Racing Thoughts

What are racing thoughts? They are a symptom of anxiety, stress, or certain mental health conditions, in which a person experiences a rapid and constant flow of thoughts that are difficult to control or slow down. These thoughts may be unrelated or challenging to follow, leading to feelings of overwhelm, restlessness, and difficulty concentrating.

Racing thoughts can interfere with work, school, or any activity that you may be doing. You can use several strategies to approach racing thoughts and cope with their impact. Firstly, it is essential to recognize when racing thoughts occur and try to identify any triggers or patterns. Two exercises that can help are meditation and yoga. They can be effective in calming the mind and slowing down racing thoughts. Talking to a mental health professional who can provide additional support and guidance can also be helpful.

Symptoms and Anger

If you are wondering how to identify if you are experiencing anxiety, the following are some common symptoms of anxiety include:

1. Excessive worry or fear about everyday situations or activities.

2. Difficulty controlling worries or irrational thoughts.

3. Restlessness or feeling on edge.

4. Muscle tension or body aches.

5. Fatigue or difficulty sleeping.

6. Difficulty concentrating or staying focused.

7. Irritability or mood swings.

8. Sweating or trembling.

9. Rapid heartbeat or shortness of breath.

Anger can also be a symptom of anxiety, but it is not a defining feature. Some people may experience anger or irritability as a response to anxiety, but others may not. It's important to recognize that everyone experiences anxiety differently, and symptoms may vary depending on the individual and the situation. Overall, monitor yourself and keep a journal. Journaling has a calming effect and can be therapeutic in many ways.

Journaling can be an effective tool for managing anxiety by helping you release your emotions, create self-awareness, help you gain a new perspective to problem solve, and reduces rumination.

Here is an in-depth look at how journaling helps:

1. Provides a release for thoughts and emotions: Writing down your thoughts and feelings can provide a cathartic release and help you process and make sense of difficult emotions.

2. Increases self-awareness: Journaling can help you identify patterns and triggers that contribute to anxiety

and track your progress in managing symptoms over time.

3. Offers a safe space for self-reflection: Journaling provides a private and non-judgmental space for self-reflection and exploration, allowing you to express yourself freely without fear of judgment or criticism.

4. Facilitates problem-solving: Writing down your concerns and anxieties can help you clarify your thoughts and identify potential solutions to problems or challenges.

5. Reduces rumination: Journaling can help break the cycle of rumination by giving you an outlet to express your thoughts and feelings rather than allowing them to loop endlessly in your mind.

In all, overcoming your anxiety is not instant. It takes daily work and practice. It requires the development of new habits and behaviors. Change is not always easy, but if you are proactive and make small adjustments to respond to the anxiety you feel positively, you can turn things around. Remember that small healthy decisions lead to massive progress over time.

Chapter 4 | Self-Care

Between all our responsibilities, it's quite easy to ignore our emotional and physical needs. Stressors are all around us, and while sometimes they can be avoided, other times they cannot. So, what do we do when we are caught in a storm where high stress and anxiety take the lead? We think about how we can better take care of ourselves.

You must take time to care for your needs—emotionally, mentally, and physically. We can do this through *self-care*. Self-care can have a positive impact on anxiety in several ways:

1. Reduces stress: Practicing self-care activities such as exercise, meditation, or spending time in nature can help reduce stress, which is a common trigger for anxiety.

2. Boosts mood: Engaging in enjoyable activities such as reading, listening to music, or spending time with loved ones can help boost mood and reduce feelings of anxiety and depression.

3. Improves physical health: Taking care of your physical health through regular exercise, healthy eating, and adequate sleep can help reduce anxiety symptoms and improve overall well-being.

4. Builds resilience: Regular self-care practices can help build resilience and strengthen coping skills, making it easier to manage stress and anxiety in challenging situations.

5. Provides a sense of control: Practicing self-care can provide a sense of control over your own well-being, which can help reduce feelings of helplessness or overwhelm associated with anxiety.

Think about what one thing you can do for yourself each day. Perhaps go for a walk, listen to music, dance, ride a bike, spend time with family or friends, exercise, and get your heart pumping. One of the best ways to care for your mind and mental health is by incorporating daily exercise into your schedule. Sure, committing to spending 45 to an hour at the gym may be difficult, but exercise can mean walking around your block, taking a dance class, signing up for a 20-minute online yoga class, or any movement that gets you up and going.

Exercise can have several positive effects on mood and mental health. Firstly, exercise releases endorphins, which are feel-good chemicals that can help reduce stress and anxiety and promote pleasure and well-being. Secondly, exercise can help regulate the levels of stress hormones in the body, such as cortisol, which can help reduce symptoms of anxiety and depression. Thirdly, regular exercise can help improve self-esteem and self-confidence, which can positively impact mood and overall well-being.

The tough part of the exercise is making it a habit, so start with ten minutes daily. Incorporate a healthy diet and plenty of rest. We live amid a hustle culture in the media that promotes working side hustles, even if it means losing sleep. But that is not healthy at all. In fact, having lousy sleep hygiene can heighten stress and further generate anxiety.

Sleep is vital for everyone, especially those struggling with anxiety. Here are a few reasons why:

- Regulates emotions: Sleep helps regulate emotions and mood, and lack of sleep can contribute to feelings of irritability, anxiety, and depression.

- Reduces stress: Getting enough sleep can help reduce stress and anxiety by giving your body and mind the time it needs to recover and recharge.

- Enhances cognitive function: Sleep is essential for cognitive function, including memory, concentration, and decision-making. Lack of sleep can impair cognitive function and exacerbate symptoms of anxiety.

- Improves physical health: Sleep is essential for physical health, including immune function, hormone regulation, and cardiovascular health. Poor sleep can contribute to a range of physical health problems that can exacerbate anxiety symptoms.

Think about how much you are sleeping. Are you exercising and moving your body? Are you taking the time to engage in self-reflection and meditation? Do you meditate or engage in an activity that calms you? All of these things matter and are part of caring for yourself.

Take good care of your mind and body because they are connected. Anxiety can impact our physical health in the following ways. Here are a few examples:

- Cardiovascular health: Anxiety can cause the release of stress hormones, such as cortisol and adrenaline, which can increase heart rate, blood pressure, and inflammation. Over time, chronic anxiety can contribute to cardiovascular problems, such as hypertension and heart disease.

- Immune function: Chronic anxiety can weaken the immune system, making it more difficult for the body to fight off infections and illnesses.

- Digestive health: Anxiety can cause digestive problems, such as stomach pain, nausea, diarrhea, and constipation. Chronic anxiety can also contribute to more serious digestive issues, such as irritable bowel syndrome (IBS).

- Respiratory health: Anxiety can cause rapid breathing and hyperventilation, leading to shortness of breath and chest pain. Chronic anxiety can also exacerbate respiratory conditions, such as asthma.

- Musculoskeletal health: Anxiety can cause tension and stiffness in the muscles and joints, leading to pain and discomfort. Chronic anxiety can also contribute to musculoskeletal conditions, such as chronic pain and fibromyalgia.

In general, anxiety can significantly impact physical health, and it's crucial to prioritize mental and physical well-being in managing anxiety. Seeking professional support and practicing healthy coping strategies, such as exercise, mindfulness, and relaxation techniques can help mitigate the physical effects of anxiety.

Chapter 5 | The Importance of Self-Compassion

Something to consider when we think about self-care is the importance of *self-compassion*. Often we are harsh with ourselves, and the inner dialogue that we have is not a positive one. We are filled with negative self-perceptions, insecurities, self-doubt, and limiting beliefs. All of which cause us an internal battle.

Interestingly, those who lack self-compassion have no problem extending compassion to others. Sometimes it could be that people are uncomfortable with self-compassion because they may think it's self-indulgent or pity. But it's not true. In fact, self-compassion may help relieve health concerns such as anxiety and insecurity.

How do you know if you lack self-compassion? Here are four signs that someone may lack self-compassion:

- Self-criticism: People who lack self-compassion often engage in harsh self-criticism, where they judge themselves harshly and hold themselves to impossibly high standards.

- Perfectionism: People who lack self-compassion may be perfectionistic, which means they have unrealistic expectations of themselves and may struggle to accept their mistakes or flaws.

- Negative self-talk: People who lack self-compassion may engage in negative self-talk, constantly berating themselves and focusing on their weaknesses and shortcomings.

- Difficulty with emotions: People who lack self-compassion may struggle to manage their emotions, as they may be overly critical of themselves and struggle to give themselves the same kindness and understanding they would offer others. They may also feel uncomfortable with vulnerability or self-disclosure.

Now that you know what it means to lack self-compassion, let's explore what it is and how we can adopt it. Self-compassion is the practice of extending the same kindness, concern, and understanding to oneself that one would offer to a good friend or loved one. It involves recognizing and accepting one's own flaws and imperfections and responding to oneself with warmth, care, and non-judgmental understanding. Self-compassion involves being mindful of one's own experiences and feelings, acknowledging them without judgment, and responding with self-kindness and support. It is a way of relating to oneself that promotes emotional well-being, resilience, and self-acceptance.

One of the best ways to develop self-compassion is by talking to yourself as though you were to someone you admire and love. In the process of speaking kindly to yourself, you will discover that you will start becoming your own ally. Think about where you spend most of your time. It's not at work or home. It's inside the walls of your mind. Therefore, the conversations you have with yourself are extremely crucial.

What you say to yourself and how you say it will dictate your mood, how you act, and your behaviors. Everything trickles down from your mind to the external world. But self-compassion does not come easy because of the things we believe about ourselves. Sometimes we may have encountered so much rejection throughout our lives that we automatically reject ourselves. Other times people around us may have uttered negative words about who we are, and over time we ended up believing those words. We begin to view ourselves from a lens of brokenness. And that's where insecurities fester.

What are the three pillars of developing self-compassion?

- Be kind to yourself: Treat yourself with kindness and understanding, just as you would a close friend or loved one. This may involve offering yourself encouragement or support, engaging in self-care activities that nurture your mind and body, or simply acknowledging your efforts and accomplishments.

- Practice self-acceptance: Recognize that imperfection and failure are normal and inevitable parts of the human experience. Rather than focusing on your shortcomings or perceived flaws, practice accepting yourself as you are, with all your strengths and weaknesses.

- Connect with others: Connect with others who are supportive and understanding, whether it's friends, family, or a support group. Being around others who are compassionate and kind can help you feel more accepted and supported.

When you are kind to yourself, you begin to care more about what you do for yourself. It becomes easier to want to establish a self-care routine because you accept yourself. When you don't like or admire yourself, you minimize your chances of living a life of happiness and fulfillment. That's when negative emotions take over because there are no boundaries.

Boundaries only exist when you love yourself enough to care about your mind, heart, and body and take the necessary steps to care for yourself. Self-compassion is the vehicle for developing self-care habits, mindfulness, exercise, and better sleep, and it will all improve the anxiety you are struggling with. Caring for yourself is important if you want to improve yourself and create a life that you are proud of. Think about the self-compassionate statements or affirmations you can tell yourself from his day forward.

Here are ten affirmations that will generate self-compassion and challenge your negative self-perceptions.

1. I am worthy of love and acceptance just as I am.

2. I am doing the best I can with the resources I have available.

3. It's okay to make mistakes. They are opportunities for growth and learning.

4. I am deserving of kindness and understanding.

5. I acknowledge my struggles and honor my journey.

6. I trust my own abilities and decisions.

7. I am not defined by my past mistakes or failures.

8. I am capable of making positive changes in my life.

9. I am allowed to set boundaries and prioritize my own needs.

10. I am grateful for the positive qualities and experiences in my life.

These affirmations can help remind you of your inherent worth, acknowledge your struggles without judgment, and encourage self-acceptance and growth. You can say these affirmations to yourself in the morning, throughout the day, or before bed to help reinforce positive self-talk and develop a more self-compassionate mindset. The more you say positive affirmations or respond positively to negative emotions, the more you reinforce good habits. Repetition is key!

When you feel out of control or may be feeling a surge of anxiety, recite the following quotes.

- "The only person you are destined to become is the person you decide to be." - Ralph Waldo Emerson

- "You are the architect of your own destiny; you are the master of your own fate; you are behind the steering wheel of your life." - Brian Tracy

- "Take responsibility for your own happiness, never put it in other people's hands." - Roy T. Bennett

- "If you don't design your own life plan, chances are you'll fall into someone else's plan. And guess what they have planned for you? Not much." - Jim Rohn

- "The greatest glory in living lies not in never falling, but in rising every time we fall." - Nelson Mandela

- "You may not control all the events that happen to you, but you can decide not to be reduced by them." - Maya Angelou

- "Be the change that you wish to see in the world." - Mahatma Gandhi

These phrases emphasize the importance of taking responsibility for your life, embracing personal growth, and being accountable for your journey. They encourage you to focus on your own goals and aspirations rather than the negative outcomes that may be happening around you. By embracing these phrases of wisdom, you can become more empowered and accountable for your life.Remember that this life that you are living only happens once. And life is too short. So, you have a choice to make. You become proactive about your emotional world and thought-life, or you allow the negative patterns to take control, leading you to suffer from mental and physical ailments.

The choice is ultimately yours!

Now that you deeply understand anxiety and its effect on you, you have work to do. Although the path ahead will not be a smooth ride, it will be worth it. Right now, think about the life you want to live. Think about what you want to feel and how you want your days to look like. Envision how you will start to approach feelings of anxiety.

Start journaling and keeping track of your daily experiences to become conscious of what you are doing, identify how you are responding, and what behaviors you need to modify. Nothing will change unless you start making the necessary behavioral changes that will automatically produce physical and emotional changes. To live the life you want to live, you must be willing to do what you have never done before.

Now that the knowledge and practical steps have been transferred to you, it's time to do your part. You can and will overcome anxiety!

Chapter 6 | Goal-Setting

Goal setting is essential to overcoming tough emotions and situations because it gives individuals a sense of purpose, direction, and motivation. When faced with challenging emotions or situations, it can be easy to feel overwhelmed and helpless, and without a clear plan or direction, it can be challenging to take action or progress. By setting goals, individuals can identify specific actions they can take to manage their emotions, improve their situation, and work toward a more positive outcome.

Setting goals can be particularly helpful in overcoming tough emotions and situations for several reasons:

1. Focus: Setting specific goals helps individuals focus their attention and energy on what is most important. This can help to reduce feelings of overwhelm and provide a sense of control over the situation.

2. Motivation: Having clear goals can motivate individuals, providing a sense of purpose and direction. When individuals have a clear idea of what they want to achieve, they are more likely to take action and persist in facing obstacles.

3. Measurable progress: Goals should be specific and measurable, which allows individuals to track their progress and celebrate their accomplishments. This can be particularly helpful in boosting motivation and confidence.

Have you ever set a goal that you achieve? Think about how you felt. The goal gave you a sense of direction, it motivated you, and once you achieved it, your confidence increased tenfold. Goal-setting can make you a fighter in the face of obstacles because you won't succumb to challenging emotions or thoughts. Your focus and motivation can help you override all the negativity. How? Your sole purpose at that moment is to reach your goal despite what's happening around you. This is a powerful mindset. In fact, in doing so, you are practicing and developing mental toughness.

And mental toughness is not only reserved for athletes. It's the kind of mindset that we can all adopt that will take us to encounter challenges with boldness and courage. Overall, goal setting can be a powerful tool for managing tough emotions and situations. By setting specific, measurable goals, individuals can focus their attention and energy, stay motivated, track their progress, and work toward a more positive outcome.

Chapter 7 | Moving Forward

The conscious mind is aware. Developing a conscious mind and mindfulness involves cultivating awareness and attention to the present moment without judgment or distraction. When you become self-aware, you begin to notice tendencies. You become in tune with your thought-life, and you sense patterns.

When you pay attention to your thoughts, you will identify two tendencies.

3. **Focus:** The mind focuses on things other than what is happening now.

4. **Evaluation:** The mind continuously evaluates our reality as good or bad.

These tendencies are part of the human experience. And quite frankly, they are inevitable. We either think about the past, the present, or the future. Thinking about the past is backward thinking, and thinking about the future is forward thinking. Both can cause anxiety. We may dive into negative emotions of regret and pain when we think about our past. When we think about the future, we may feel fear and anxiety because it's unknown. We may even think about adverse outcomes or all the bad turns our life can take.

However, when we focus on our present, we eliminate the automatic effort to judge things in the past or future. Mindfulness is the anecdote to shift our focus from the past and future and constantly evaluate things as negative or good. We must simply live in the moment. It abolishes both tendencies.

Mindfulness is much more than acknowledging what you are doing at the moment. It's about diving deeper and being intentional. It's about cultivating a connection with our present experience.

Here are some strategies for becoming more conscious and developing mindfulness:

7. Practice mindfulness meditation: One of the most effective ways to cultivate mindfulness is through regular meditation. Mindfulness meditation involves focusing on the present moment, such as your breath or bodily sensations, and noticing when your mind wanders without judgment.

8. Pay attention to your senses: Another way to become more conscious is to focus your attention on your senses. For example, when you're eating, pay attention to your food's taste, texture, and aroma. When you're outside, notice the sights, sounds, and smells around you. When you are becoming frustrated or angry, think about the root cause of your anger. Do you feel a lack of control? Do you feel helpless? What is triggering your anger? And then, instead of resisting, allow things to play out. Resistance to situations only increases frustration.

9. Take breaks from technology: Technology can be a major distraction that pulls us away from the present moment. To become more conscious, try taking breaks from technology, such as turning off your phone or computer for a few hours each day.

10. Practice gratitude: Focusing on what you're grateful for can help you become more conscious of the positive aspects of your life. Take time each day to reflect on what you're thankful for- a supportive friend, a beautiful sunset, or a favorite hobby.

11. Engage in mindful activities: Engaging in activities that require focused attention, such as yoga, tai chi, or painting, can help you develop mindfulness and become more conscious.

12. Be present with others: When you're with other people, make an effort to be fully present and engaged in the conversation. Avoid distractions such as phones or other devices, and focus on actively listening and responding to the person in front of you.

Becoming more conscious and developing mindfulness takes time and practice, but with consistent effort, it is possible to cultivate greater awareness and presence in your daily life.